Shema AYADI

Eating and lifestyle habits in NAFLD

Shema AYADI

Eating and lifestyle habits in NAFLD

Imprint
Any brand names and product names mentioned in this book are subject to trademark, brand or patent protection and are trademarks or registered trademarks of their respective holders. The use of brand names, product names, common names, trade names, product descriptions etc. even without a particular marking in this work is in no way to be construed to mean that such names may be regarded as unrestricted in respect of trademark and brand protection legislation and could thus be used by anyone.

Cover image: www.ingimage.com

This book is a translation from the original published under ISBN 978-620-6-68907-2.

Publisher:
Sciencia Scripts
is a trademark of
Dodo Books Indian Ocean Ltd. and OmniScriptum S.R.L publishing group

120 High Road, East Finchley, London, N2 9ED, United Kingdom
Str. Armeneasca 28/1, office 1, Chisinau MD-2012, Republic of Moldova, Europe
Printed at: see last page
ISBN: 978-620-6-33075-2

TABLE OF CONTENTS

INTRODUCTION

These days, food hygiene and the excessive consumption of fatty foods are a hot topic. Indeed, according to the World Health Organization (WHO), inadequate nutrition is a major risk factor in the development of several chronic diseases, such as cardiovascular disease, cancer, diabetes mellitus and obesity. A diet rich in products with a high sugar and salt content is the dietary disorder most often incriminated in the development of these pathologies. The food industry, a sedentary lifestyle and a fast-paced urban lifestyle all play their part in the development and perpetuation of these unsuitable eating habits, endangering the health of the populations concerned. One of the chronic diseases caused by a diet too rich in added sugars is non-alcoholic fatty liver disease (NAFLD).Non-alcoholic fatty liver disease (NAFLD) is a liver disorder secondary to intrahepatocyte fat accumulation (around 5% of liver volume) in the absence of alcohol consumption and specific pathologies[1]. It is a pathology with different stages of severity depending on the degree of histological damage. Indeed, hepatic inflammation is not constant, and its presence, translated histologically by the presence of hepatocyte ballooning and an inflammatory infiltrate, defines non-alcoholic steatohepatitis (NASH)[1], observed in around 20% of NAFLD[2]. The acute inflammation seen in NASH can progress to hepatic fibrosis ranging from minimal fibrosis to full-blown cirrhosis, with the risk of developing hepatocellular carcinoma[1].

Metabolically speaking, sugar is converted into fat by the liver for storage when needed. But when the intake of sugars and fats is too high, the liver produces and stores excess fat, leading to hepatic steatosis. Clinically, apart from cirrhosis and advanced liver fibrosis, the spectrum of NAFLD diseases is often asymptomatic, often discovered incidentally on abdominal imaging data[3]. Ultrasound remains the most widely used non-invasive examination for diagnosing hepatic steatosis with a sensitivity of 60-94% and a specificity of 84-.95%[4] Similarly, the diagnosis may be made in the presence of non-specific symptoms such as fatigue with reduced physical capacity, asthenia or pain in the right hypochondrium. Finally, the diagnosis may be made as part of an investigation into hepatic cytolysis, or when the physician suspects liver damage in the presence of risk factors such as obesity, dyslipidemia or diabetes mellitus[5].

NAFLD is a major cause of liver disease worldwide. Indeed, the global prevalence of NAFLD is 25.24%, affecting one in four people worldwide, with the highest prevalence in the Middle East and South America, and the lowest in Africa[6]. Similarly, NASH is currently the 1st cause of chronic liver disease and the 3rd leading cause of liver transplantation in the United States[7].

Management of this pathology, supported by pathophysiological data, relies largely on identifying lifestyle habits and inadequate nutrition, in order to propose the necessary corrections. Thus, the aim of our study was to:

Describe dietary and lifestyle habits in patients with non-alcoholic fatty liver disease.

METHODS

1. Type of study

We conducted a descriptive cross-sectional study in the hepato-gastroenterology department of Charles Nicolle Hospital, during the period from November 17, 2022 to February 03, 2023.

2. Population studied

Our study included all patients with non-alcoholic fatty liver presenting to the outpatient department of the Hepato-Gastroenterology Service at Charles Nicolle Hospital during the study period.

2.1. Inclusion criteria

Patients included:

- Having non-alcoholic fatty liver diagnosed on the abdominal ultrasound data.

- Over 18 years of age.

2.2. Non inclusion criteria

Patients were not included:

- With secondary hepatic steatosis (alcohol, viral hepatitis, etc.) hypothyroidism, medication ...)

- Patients who did not consent to participate in the study.

3. Methods

3.1. Data collection :

Patient data were collected using a pre-established information sheet. We noted the following characteristics:

3.1.1. Characteristics socio-demographic

The patient's age, sex, place of residence, marital status, level of education, professional status, socio-economic conditions and housing were recorded at the start of the interview.

3.1.2. Personal history

We recorded personal histories of diabetes mellitus, hypercholesterolemia, hypertriglyceridemia, arterial hypertension, hypothyroidism, hyperthyroidism, coronary insufficiency, parity, breastfeeding and menopause. Similarly, we specified the following lifestyle habits: the existence or not of active or weaned smoking, occasional alcohol consumption and physical activity.

Physical activity has been described as :

✓ Absent or irregular: if the patient performed little or no activity physical (<1 time/week).

✓ Average: if the patient performed physical activity once or twice a week.

✓ Good: if the patient was physically active more than three times a week.

3.1.3. Examination physical

The following data were collected for each patient:
✓ Weight, height and waist circumference

✓ Body mass index (BMI): Calculated by dividing weight (in kilograms) by the square of height (in meters) (Kg/m²).

✓ Dentition status: patients' dentition was classified as "good" if they had dentition that could ensure adequate chewing of food, and "bad" if they had dentition that could not ensure adequate chewing of food.

3.1.4. Biological examinations

We recorded the most recent biology data, no more than 06 months old from the date of inclusion in the study. Biological parameters were taken from the patient's medical record. These parameters were as follows: Fasting blood glucose, Triglycerides, Total cholesterol, LDL cholesterol, HDL cholesterol, Uric acid, Platelets, AST, ALT, GGT, PAL.

3.1.5. Definition of metabolic syndrome

We noted the presence or absence of metabolic syndrome in our patients. We based our definition of metabolic syndrome on that of the IDF[8].According to this definition, an individual is a carrier of this syndrome when he or she presents three or more of the following five criteria:

1) Abdominal obesity, estimated by a waist circumference ≥ 94cm in men and ≥80cm for women.
2) Elevation of fasting triglyceridemia ≥ 1.50 g/l (1.7mmol/L) or treatment.
3) A reduction in HDL cholesterol < 0.4 g/l (1.03mmol/l) in men and < 0.5 g/l (1.29mmol/L) in women.

4) An increase in blood pressure ≥ 130/85 mm Hg or treatment.

5) A fasting blood glucose level ≥ 1 g/l (5.6mmol/l) or treatment.

3.1.6. Hepatic fibrosis stage

The stage of hepatic fibrosis was determined by :

✓ The FIB-4 score is calculated using the following formula: FIB-4 = (Age x ASAT) / (Platelets x √ [ALAT])

The absence of severe hepatic fibrosis was defined by a score of FIB-4<1.3

✓ Liver elasticity value by Fibroscan if performed.

Minimal to moderate hepatic fibrosis was defined by hepatic elastometry < 8Kpa[9].

3.1.7. Eating habits

For each patient, we specified whether or not they fasted during Ramadan, outside Ramadan or intermittently, whether or not they had a history of following a ketogenic or Mediterranean diet, and whether or not they chewed their food well. We also specified where meals were taken (home, restaurant, workplace).

3.1.8. Food survey

We carried out a dietary survey to assess patients' food consumption and eating habits.To do this, we used the food history method. This is a qualitative and quantitative estimate of a person's nutritional intake, based on the time of day at which the meal was eaten, the nature of the food consumed, its quantity, frequency of consumption, and method of preparation.To estimate the approximate quantities consumed, we used a manual listing photographed portions (Livret des portions alimentaires -

Institut de Nutrition de Tunis)[10].Finally, to synthesize the information gathered, by transforming the quantities of food consumed daily into nutrients, we entered each patient's dietary surveys into Bilnut software version 2.01, in order to obtain an estimate of spontaneous nutritional intakes.The summary of spontaneous nutritional intakes of micro- and macronutrients includes the following elements:

- Total daily calorie intake.

- Protein, carbohydrate and fat intake, and their daily distribution.

- The breakdown of lipid intake into saturated (SFA), monounsaturated (MUFA) and polyunsaturated (PUFA) fatty acids.

- Cholesterol, sucrose and fiber intake.

- Vitamins: Vitamin C, Vitamin E, Vitamin B9, Vitamin B1.

- Trace elements and minerals: iron, calcium, potassium, sodium, magnesium, zinc, phosphorus.

- **Estimated total energy requirements :**

We estimated the energy requirements of each patient according to the following formula:

DET = MB x NAP

So to determine this formula we calculated the basic metabolism (BM) in kcal according to the formula of Black et al and we estimated the physical activity level (PAL) (according to EFSA NDA Panel, 2013)[11].

3.1.9. Consumption frequency questionnaire

In addition, we chose to carry out a questionnaire on the frequency of consumption of certain foods, beverages and cooking methods (number of times per week, month). For each food, drink or cooking method on the list, the patient has indicated his or her usual consumption.

3.2. Statistical analysis of data

Data were entered and analyzed using Excel 2019 software.
We have calculated :

• Absolute frequencies and relative frequencies (percentages) for categorical variables.

• Means, standard deviations and extreme values for quantitative variables.

3.3. Search bibliography

The bibliographic search was carried out via the following search engines: Pubmed, Science Direct and Google Scholar.The keywords used, in French, were: Stéatose hépatique non-alcoolique, habitudes alimentaires, habitudes de vie, and in English: Non-alcoholic fatty liver disease, dietary habits, lifestyles.

3.4. Ethical considerations

For each patient, we explained the purpose and modalities of the study in order to obtain consent. An informed consent form in Arabic was signed by the patient before inclusion in the study. Consenting individuals were interviewed discreetly, using simple, explicit language.Patient data are processed and stored as follows anonymously.

RESULTS

1. General characteristics of the population studied

In our study, we included 42 patients with non-alcoholic hepatic steatosis.

1.1.Characteristics socio-demographic

1.1.1. Age

Patients ranged in age from 29 to 70 years, with an average age of 56.29 ±8.65 years.The majority of the population (45%) was aged between 60 and 70. The distribution of patients by age group is illustrated in figure 1.

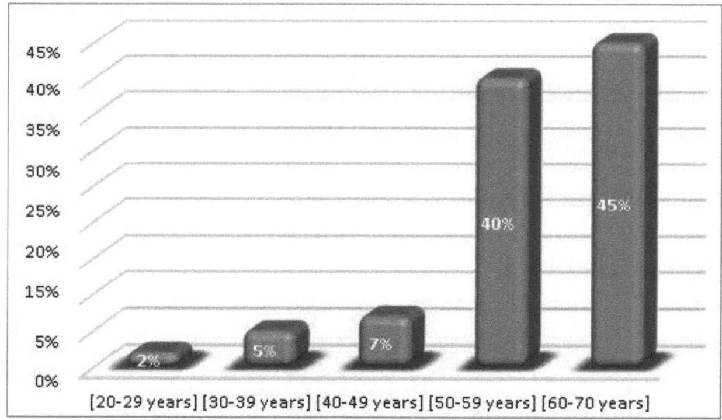

Figure 1: Age distribution of patients

1.1.2. Gender

The patients were predominantly female, with an M/F sex ratio of 0.4. The distribution of patients by sex is shown in figure 2.

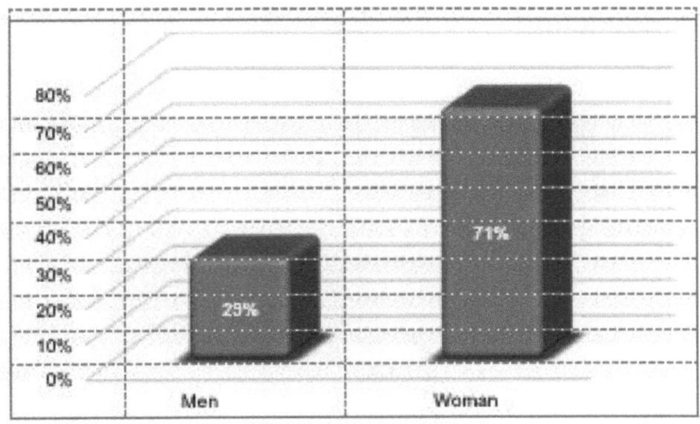

Figure 2: Distribution of patients by gender

1.1.3. Marital status :

Married status was the most common marital status among our patients. The distribution of patients by marital status is shown in figure 3.

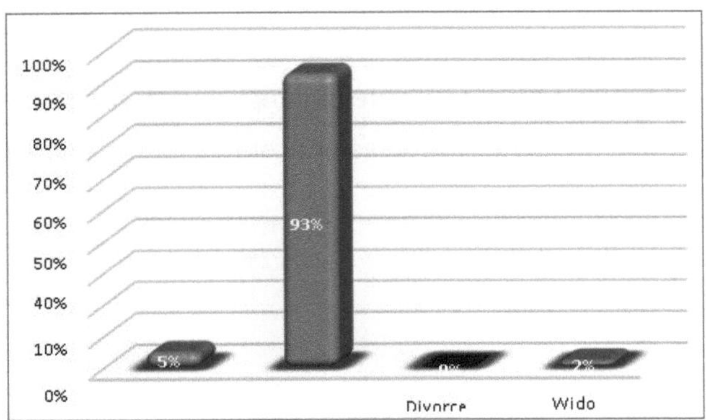

Figure 3:Distribution of patients by marital status

1.1.4. Level of education

The majority of our patients (64%) had a low level of education (no schooling).schooling or primary school level). The patients' level of education is shown in figure 4.

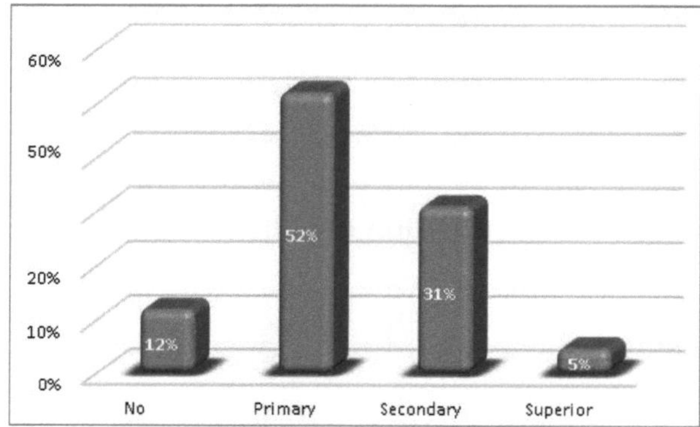

Figure 4: Population distribution by education level

1.1.5. Status professional

The majority of patients (62%) were unemployed, housewife or retired). The distribution of patients by professional status is illustrated in figure 5.

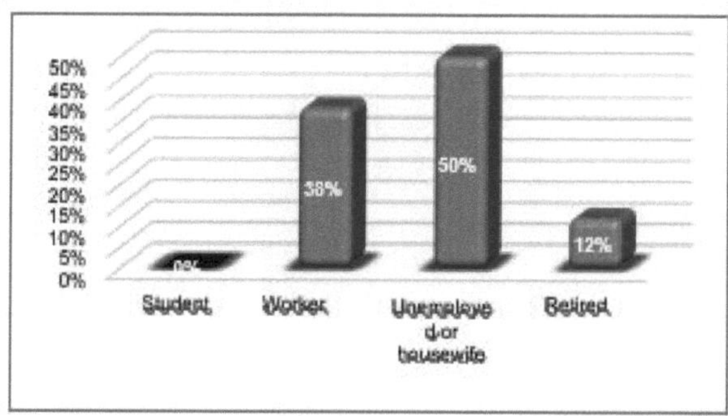

Figure 5: Distribution of patients by professional status

1.1.6. Level socioeconomic

The majority of our patients were of average socioeconomic status. The distribution of patients by socio-economic level is shown in figure 6.

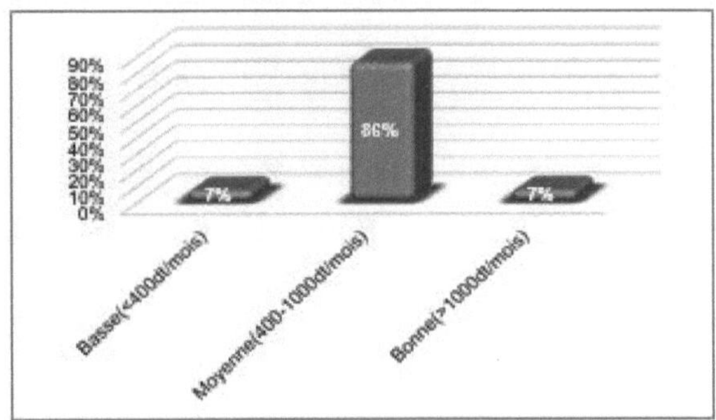

Figure 6: Distribution of patients by socio-economic level

1.1.7. Location

All patients lived in urban areas.

1.1.8. Housing

The entire population lived in families.

1.2. History

1.2.1. Medical

A personal history of hypertension and dyslipidemia was the most common.in our population (48% respectively). The personal history of the study population is illustrated in figure 7.

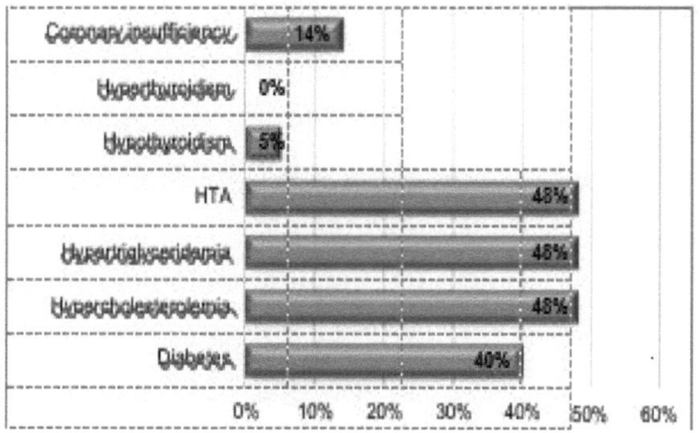

Figure 7: Population distribution by personal history

1.2.2. Gyneco-obstetrics

• Parity :

The majority of our patients (85%) had a history of parity. Multiparity (≥4 parities) was noted in 41% of our patients.

• Breast-feeding

The notion of breast-feeding was found in 24 patients (80%). The duration of breastfeeding varied from 6 to 24 months.

• Menopause

Menopause was observed in 87% of included patients.

1.2.3. Lifestyle

• Tobacco consumption

The majority of patients did not smoke (90%). The distribution of patients by smoking status is shown in figure 8.

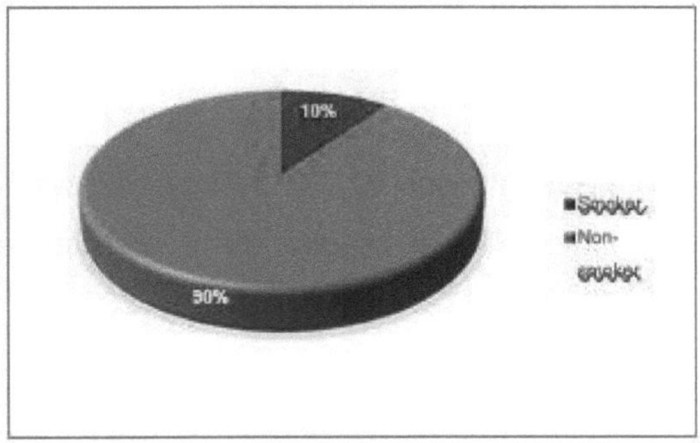

Figure 8: Distribution of patients by smoking status

• Occasional alcohol consumption

Occasional alcohol consumption was noted in 5% of our population.

• Physical activity

More than half the patients were sedentary or practised sport irregularly (55%).Figure 9 illustrates the distribution of patients according to their level of physical activity.

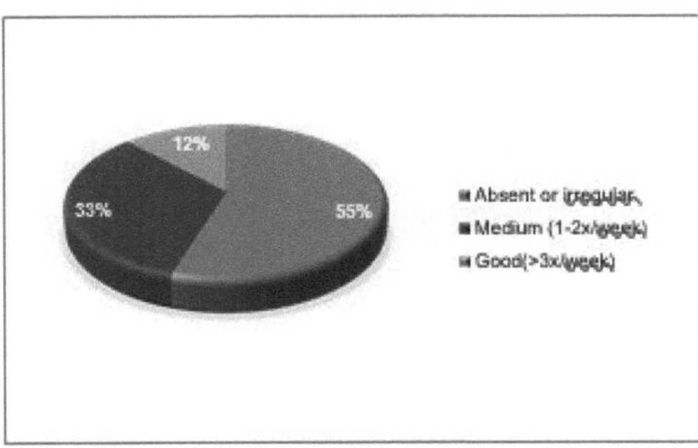

Figure 9: Distribution of patients by physical activity level

1.3.Examination data physical

1.3.1. Anthropometric measurements

The mean BMI of our patients was 30.79± 3.98 kg/m2, with 45% overweight and 55% obese.The averageanthropometricparameters ofour population are shown in Table I.

Table I: Anthropometric parameters

Parameters	Mean± standard deviation
Current weight (kg)	80,01± 10 ,79
Size (cm)	161,38± 9,16
BMI (kg/m2)	30,79± 3,98
Waist circumference (cm)	102,05± 11,29

1.3.2. Condition of teeth

The condition of the population's teeth was judged to be good in 2/3 of our patients (Figure 10).

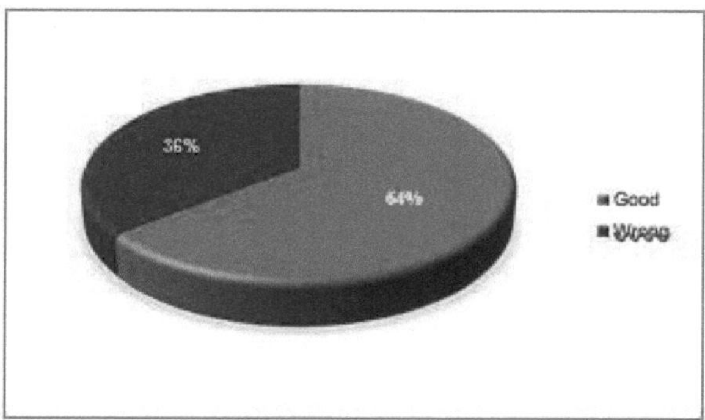

Figure 10: Distribution of patients by dentition status

2. Characteristics of liver damage

2.1. Characteristics

Hyperglycemia, hypertriglyceridemia and hypercholesterolemia were observed in 56%, 42% and 34% of our patients respectively.The majority of patients (71%) had low HDL cholesterol levels.Cytolysis (increased ASAT and/or ALAT) was present in 14% of patients. The results of the biological parameters of our population are shown in Table II.

Table II: Average biological parameters collected

Parameters	Mean ± standard deviation
GAJ (mmol/L)	7,56± 4,14
TG (mmol/L)	1,66± 0,7
Cholesterol (mmol/L)	4,99± 1,7
LDL cholesterol (mmol/L)	2,23± 0,79
HDL cholesterol (mmol/L)	1,15± 0,32
Uric acid (mg/L)	34,94± 9,15
Platelets(x10^3/mm3)	288,63± 73,64
AST (UI/L)	21,95± 9,55
ALAT (UI/L)	23,8± 11,73
GGT (UI/L)	39,94± 29,65
PAL (IU/L)	87,44± 38,92

2.2.Associated metabolic syndrome

In our population, the majority of patients (69%) had a metabolic syndrome.The distribution of our population according to metabolic syndrome is illustrated in figure 11.

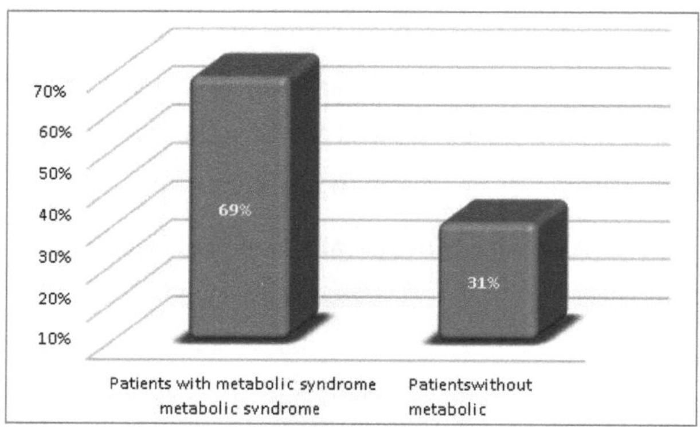

Figure 11: Distribution of patients according to metabolic syndrome

2.3. Hepatic fibrosis

The majority of patients (80%) had a FIB-4 score of less than 1.3, excluding severe hepatic fibrosis.Similarly, 83% of patients had hepatic elastometry < 8Kpa, consistent with minimal to moderate hepatic fibrosis. The means of the patients' fibrosis diagnostic parameters are shown in Table III.

Table III: Average fibrosis diagnostic parameters

Parameters	Mean ± standard deviation
FIB-4	0,97± 0,49
Fibroscan	6,03± 2,53

3. Eating habits and survey

3.1. Eating habits

All patients were not practicing intermittent fasting or following a ketogenic diet.Table IV shows the percentage distribution of patients according to certain dietary habits.

Table IV: Distribution of patients according to certain eating habits

Variables		Corresponding percentage
Ramadan fasting	Yes	86%
	No	14%
Fasting at outside of ramadan	Yes	38%
	No	62%
Intermittent fasting	Yes	0%
	No	100%
History of ketogenic diet	Yes	0%
	No	100%
History of education on the Mediterranean diet	Yes	57%
	No	43%
Good mastication of food	Yes	60%
	No	40%
Meal location	House	100%
	Restaurant	14%
	Place of work	10%

3.2.Results of the food survey

3.2.1. Total energy expenditure and intake

Spontaneous caloric intake in our population (3386.14 kcal) was higher than energy requirements (2490.14 kcal).The averages of patients' theoretical energy requirements and their spontaneous caloric intake are presented in Table V.

Table V: Patients' average theoretical energy requirements and spontaneous calorie intake

Variables	Mean ± standard deviation
Metabolism of metabolism (according black et al formula)	1472,1± 179,68
NAP	1,69± 0,1
Expenses energy total (in kcal)	2490,14± 346,96
Total energy intake (in kcal)	3386,14± 785,7

3.2.2. Intake of macronutrients

the majority of participants had a high-carbohydrate (>5g/kg/Pi), high-fat (>1g/kg/Pi) and high-protein (>1g/kg/Pi) diet, in line with FAO and WHO recommendations[12]. Table VI shows the average spontaneous macronutrient intakes of our patients.

Table VI: Average spontaneous macronutrient intake

Macronutrients	Mean ± standard deviation
Protein (g/d)	78,84± 24,42
Fat (g/d)	80,54± 32,17
Carbohydrates (g/d)	336,61± 127,74
Grams of protein / kg ideal weight	1,36± 0,41
Gram fat / kg ideal weight	1,4± 0,58
Grams of carbohydrate / kg ideal weight	5,86± 2,22

3.2.3. Contribution of SFA, MUFA and PUFA

SFA, MUFA and PUFA intakes as a percentage of total energy intake exceed the standards set by the Swiss Federal Office of Public Health (FOPH) and the European Society of Cardiology (ESC):

• SFA < 7% TEA ;

• AGMI : 15% AET ;

• AGPI : 6-8 % AET ;

Patients' spontaneous intakes of SFAs, MUFAs and PUFAs are presented in Table VII.

Tabl VII: Spontaneous intakes of SFAs, MUFAs and PUFAs

Nutrients	Mean ± standard deviation
SFA (% TEA)	23± 5,5
MUFA (% TEA)	48,7± 12,67
PUFAS (% TEA)	28,31± 11,87

3.2.4. Cholesterol, sugar and fiber content

The average cholesterol intake found in our patients was in line with ANSES recommendations.On the other hand, average sugar intake (sucrose) exceeded ANSES recommendations. And average fiber intake was below ANSES recommendations. Average cholesterol, sugar (sucrose) and fiber intakes for the population are shown in Table VIII.

Table VIII: Cholesterol, sugar and fiber intake

Nutrients	The inputs recommended : ANSES	Mean ± standard deviation
Cholesterol (mg/d)	< 300	115,33± 119,71
Sugar (sucrose) (g/d)	< 100	124,54± 39,68
Fiber (g/d)	30	25,6± 11,18

3.2.5. Micronutrient intake

The results showed that the average intake of vitamin B9, calcium, magnesium and potassium was insufficient in relation to ANSES recommendations.Average micronutrient intakes (vitamins, minerals and trace elements) are shown in Table IX.

Table IX: Micronutrient intake

Micronutrients	The inputs recommended : ANSES	Mean ± standard deviation
Vitamin B1 (µg/d)	0,1	0,96± 0,58
Vitamin B9 (µg/d)	330	238,55± 114,3
Vitamin C (mg/d)	110	216,19± 143,12
Vitamin E (mg/d)	Men:10; women: 9	12,11± 8,93
Iron (mg/d)	Men:11; women: 11-16	16,9± 5,86
Calcium (mg/d)	950-1000	584,1± 206,01
Sodium (mg/d)	1500	1490,52± 847,06
Magnesium (mg/d)	Men:380-420 ; women: 300-360	232,4± 131,5
Potassium (mg/d)	3500	2066,86± 904,5
Zinc (mg/d)	Men:5-14; women: 7.5-11	72,67± 113,24
Phosphorus (mg/d)	550-700	722,69± 310,7

3.3.Frequencies consumption

According to the food frequency questionnaire, we have noted that :

- More than ¾ of the population consumed white sugar, white bread and fruits high in fructose such as watermelons, grapes and apricots on a daily basis.

- Around half of our patients consumed fruits daily, which are also very rich in fructose, such as pears, figs, dates and bananas.

- However, we also ensured that none of the patients decaffeinated coffee and symbiotic yoghurt.

DISCUSSION

In this study, we present a single-center, cross-sectional, descriptive study of the dietary and lifestyle habits of patients with non-alcoholic fatty liver disease.We included 42 patients with a mean age of 56.29 ± 8.65 years and a sex ratio M/F equal to 0.4. The majority of women included were postmenopausal (87%) with a history of parity and breastfeeding in 85% and 80% respectively. Metabolic syndrome was observed in 69% of our patients. In addition, the majority of our population (80%) did not have advanced liver fibrosis.The main dietary habits described in our population were: a caloric diet, a diet rich in carbohydrates, lipids, proteins, SFAs, MUFAs, PUFAs, sugar (sucrose), fruits rich in fructose and a diet low in fiber. The majority of patients were Ramadan fasters. No patient practised intermittent fasting during the rest of the year. The main lifestyle habit of our population was a sedentary lifestyle. However, smoking was not frequently found in our population.

The highlights of our study are :
- This work includes patients with the various stages of NAFLD, not just those with simple hepatic steatosis.
- Our study focused on eating habits, taking into account the socio-cultural context of our country.
- We also studied patients' lifestyle habits, which are often poorly evaluated in the literature.

However, our work has certain limitations:
- This is mainly due to the relatively small size of the study population, explained by the limited recruitment time and the short study period. In fact, increasing the number of participants would have provided a larger sample size, increasing the reliability of the results.

- Patients were recruited from a public hospital. As a result, some of the more affluent social classes, preferring to consult in the private sector, could not be included in our sample. This could represent a selection bias. Non-alcoholic fatty liver disease (NAFLD) is a liver disease characterized by an excessive accumulation of fat in the liver (steatosis), in the absence of excessive alcohol consumption. According to a study by the European Society for the Study of the Liver (EASL), the prevalence of NAFLD is rising steadily, and is estimated at around 25% of the world's population[13]. The pathogenesis of NAFLD is complex and not yet fully understood. Several factors are involved, including an imbalance in the excessive intake of fatty acids from the diet, disruption of the gut-liver axis due to dysbiosis, release of fatty acids from adipose tissue, excessive fat production by the liver, and reduced elimination and oxidation of fatty acids. This imbalance leads to an accumulation of lipids, mainly in the form of triglycerides, in liver cells, which then triggers inflammation and fibrosis via increased cytokines (TNF-α, IL6, IL-8, IL1β) and oxidative stress[14,15]. Triglyceride accumulation in the liver interferes with insulin signaling pathways within cells, leading to insulin resistance and increased hepatic glucose and triglyceride production[16,17]. Another pathophysiological mechanism observed in NAFLD is the disruption of mitochondrial biogenesis and function, contributing to insulin resistance and fat accumulation in the liver[18-20].

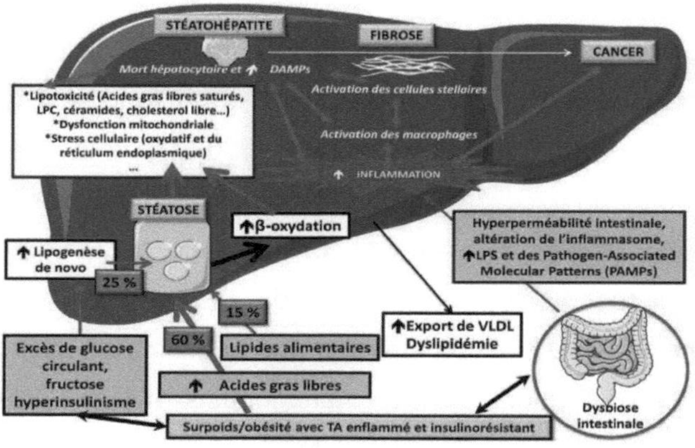

Figure 12: Schematic representation of the development of steatosis and metabolic steatohepatitis (NASH)[20].

NAFLD comprises a broad spectrum of liver disorders, with two main histological forms: Non Fatty Liver Disease or NAFL and Non Alcoholic Steato Hepatitis or NASH. NAFL is characterized by simple fat accumulation with at least 5% steatosis, but little or no inflammation and hepatocellular damage [21]. NASH is a more active form of NAFLD characterized by extensive inflammation, swelling and fibrosis, which can progress to advanced fibrosis, cirrhosis and hepatocellular carcinoma[21].

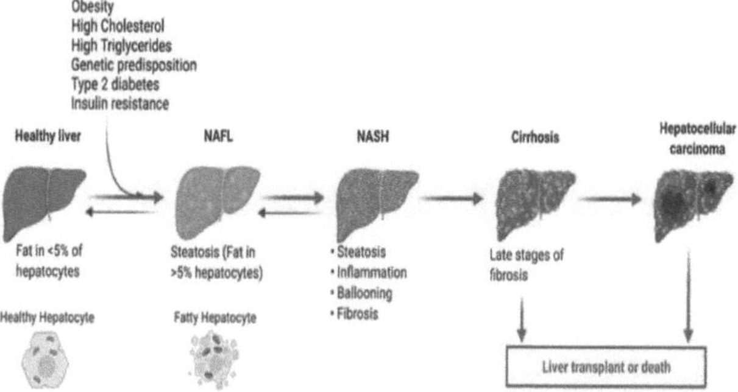

Figure 13: The NAFLD spectrum[22].

1. General characteristics of the population

1.1.Characteristics socio-demographic

1.1.1. Age

The mean age of our patients was 56.29 ± 8.65 years, with 45% between 60 and 70 years of age. Indeed, a cross-sectional study conducted in Turkey revealed variations in the prevalence of non-alcoholic fatty liver disease according to patient age. The results showed that the mean age of the population was 43.67 ±11.83 years, and the lowest prevalence of NAFLD was observed in patients aged under 30, with a rate of 23.0%. In contrast, prevalence was highest in patients over 50, reaching 65.6%. Patients aged between 30 and 40 had a prevalence of 38.7%, while in those aged between 40 and 50, the prevalence was 52.6%. In addition, the study also revealed a significant increase in the severity of hepatic steatosis with age[23]. On the other hand, another study by Hu et al, which included 7152 adults, showed that the mean age of subjects with NAFLD was 46.82 ± 13.50 years, and 40.29 ± 14.76 years in those without NAFLD. Moreover, the prevalence of NAFLD increased with age, with the highest prevalence (54%) in the 50-65 age group[24].

1.1.2. Gender

Female predominance was noted in our population. However, in a Japanese study conducted over 12 years, the average prevalence of hepatic steatosis in men was 26%, double that observed in women (13%)[25]. In another study by Chen et al. the authors found that men were more likely to develop hepatic steatosis than women, but that women with hepatic steatosis tended to have a more severe form of the disease[26].The discrepancy between our results and those of the literature could be explained by a selection bias and the small size of our sample.

1.1.3. Status marital

The majority of our patients (93%) were married. This result is in line with a Korean study which showed that 74.93 ± 1.75% of NAFLD patients were married[27]. In addition, a study by Motamed et al found that marriage is a potential risk factor for NAFLD [28]. This could be explained by a change in eating habits after marriage.

1.1.4. Level of education

The majority of our patients (64%) had a low level of education (no schooling or primary school level). This is in agreement with the results of an American study [29]which reported that individuals with a higher level of education had a lower risk of NAFLD than those with a lower level of education. This could be explained by the fact that patients with a good level of education are more interested in their health, with particular attention paid to their diet and physical image. Better financial access to a varied and balanced diet could also explain these results.

1.1.5. Status professional

The majority of patients (62%) had no professional activity (unemployed, housewife or pensioner), a finding consistent with that of a study carried out in Iran, which showed that 50.4% of NAFLD patients were unemployed[30]. Unemployed status would, in fact, encourage an imbalance in diet (insufficient consumption of fruit and fish, non-use of quality vegetable oil, etc.) due to financial incapacity.

1.1.6. Level socioeconomic

The majority of our patients were of average socioeconomic status. Indeed, a study of the correlation between income and non-alcoholic fatty liver disease in a Chinese population[31], found that as income levels increased, so did the prevalence of NAFLD. This is at odds with our results, and would be mainly due to the variability of dietary habits between the populations studied. In ours, the low level Socioeconomic is most likely linked to unemployment and low levels of education, justifying our results.

1.1.7. Location

In our study, all patients lived in urban areas. In a Chinese study [32], the prevalence of NAFLD (21.83%) in urban areas was almost equal to that (20.43%) in rural areas.

1.1.8. Housing

The entire population lived in families. This notion has not been studied in other works.

1.2. History

1.2.1. Medical

A personal history of hypertension and dyslipidemia was the most common.in our population (48% respectively). A French study[33] showed that in people with NAFLD, the prevalence of dyslipidemia was estimated at 41-69%, and that of hypertension at 39%. Similarly, diabetes was present in 40% of the population studied. A Tunisian study including 113 patients with NAFLD also showed that type 2 diabetes was present in 42.5% of these patients[34].Coronary heart disease was present in 14% of the population. The study by Armandi and Bugianesi found that non-alcoholic fatty liver disease is associated with an increased prevalence of cardiovascular disease, including hypertension, arrhythmias, atherosclerosis, coronary artery disease and heart failure[35].This reinforces what we already know about NAFLD, which goes beyond liver damage to form part of a multisystem metabolic disorder: the metabolic syndrome, with its various complications, in particular cardiovascular complications.

1.2.2. Gyneco-obstetrics

• Parity

Most of our patients (85%) had a history of parity, 41% of whom were multiparous. This finding is consistent with that of an American study that explored the association between parity and the prevalence of NAFLD in the US population, and reported that parity, regardless of the number of children or age at first birth, was associated with an increased risk of NAFLD[36]. This could be explained by the weight gain induced by pregnancy, which increases the risk of secondarily developing NAFLD.

• Breast-feeding

Of the patients included in the study, 24 (80%) reported breastfeeding. The duration of breastfeeding varied from 6 months to 24 months. In contrast, a study of 6,893 Korean women aged 30-50 who participated in the Korean National Health and Nutrition Examination Survey were assessed for the association between breastfeeding and NAFLD. The results of this study showed that there was a significant association between breastfeeding and a reduced risk of NAFLD in women compared with those who had not breastfed. Moreover, a longer duration of breastfeeding was associated with a greater reduction in the risk of NAFLD[37]. This protective role of breastfeeding could be explained by the known benefit of breastfeeding in reducing the onset of diabetes and metabolic syndrome. The effect on the occurrence of NAFLD could thus be deduced. However, the exact mechanism behind the protective effect of breastfeeding needs further study. This effect does not appear to be present in our population, most probably due to the multifactorial nature of NAFLD genesis.

• Menopause

Menopause was observed in 87% of included patients. These results concur with those of a cross-sectional study conducted in north-eastern Germany. This study included 808 women aged between 40 and 59, and revealed a significant association between menopausal status and the presence of hepatic steatosis in women. Postmenopausal women were more likely to develop hepatic steatosis than those who were still menstruating[38], and this was probably due to the loss of the known protective effect of estrogen on the genesis of NAFLD.

1.2.3. Lifestyle

• Tobacco consumption

The majority of patients did not smoke (90%). While the results of a Korean cohort study showed a positive association between tobacco consumption and the risk of developing NAFLD. People who smoked were more likely to develop NAFLD than non-smokers[39], secondary to smoking-induced increases in pro-inflammatory cytokines, chronic hypoxemia and insulin resistance.

• Occasional alcohol consumption

Occasional alcohol consumption was noted in 5% of our population. The study by Jarvis H et al, which was a systematic review of longitudinal observational cohort studies, concluded that there was limited and conflicting evidence regarding the effect of moderate alcohol consumption on the progression of liver disease in patients with NAFLD. Some studies suggested an association between moderate alcohol consumption and more rapid disease progression, while others found no significant association [40].

• Physical activity

More than half the patients were sedentary or practised sport irregularly (55%).Our results are comparable to those presented in the study by Hallsworth et al. These authors revealed that NAFLD patients had higher levels of sedentary behaviors, measured using physical activity recording devices, compared to healthy individuals. In addition, NAFLD patients were less physically active than participants in the control group[41]. This underlines the already known role of a sedentary lifestyle in the genesis of NAFLD.

1.3. Examination data physical

1.3.1. Anthropometric measurements

The mean BMI of our patients was 30.79± 3.98 kg/m2, with 45% overweight and 55% obese.A study carried out in Iran on 206 patients with non-alcoholic fatty liver disease found that the mean BMI was31±1.5kg/m2 and also showed that previous studies estimated that nearly 30% to 100% of these patients were obese[42].Moreover, another study in Croatia found that up to 80% of NAFLD patients are obese[43].

Moreover, the mean weight in our population was 80.01± 10.79 kg. Indeed, Shen et al showed in a study of 146 patients with biopsy evidence of NAFLD that the mean weight of these patients was 74.5 ± 14.8 kg [44]. Furthermore, in our study the mean waist circumference was 102.05± 11.29 cm. This result coincides with that of a study carried out in Liverpool, which revealed that waist circumference was high in subjects with NAFLD, with a mean of 108.6± 9[45].Furthermore, Cabrera et al found in their study that waist circumference was significantly associated with an increased risk of NAFLD in older adults in Guayaquil. An increase in waist circumference was associated with a greater prevalence of NAFLD, independently of BMI. This suggests that obesity Abdominal, as measured by waist circumference, may be an important risk factor for the development of NAFLD in the elderly[46].

1.3.2. Condition of teeth

The condition of the population's teeth was judged to be good in 2/3 of our patients. This parameter had not been studied in the literature. We opted to study this parameter in order to investigate a possible association between poor mastication due to poor oral condition and the onset of NAFLD. However, this association did not appear to occur.

2. Characteristics of liver damage

2.1.Features

Hyperglycemia, hypertriglyceridemia and hypercholesterolemia were observed in 56%, 42% and 34% of our patients respectively.The majority of patients (71%) had low HDL cholesterol levels. Cytolysis (increased ASAT and/or ALAT) was present in 14% of patients. Indeed, several studies have reported alterations in biological parameters in individuals with non-alcoholic fatty liver disease (NAFLD). Elevated levels of glucose, triglycerides, total cholesterol, AST and ALT were frequently observed in NAFLD patients compared to healthy subjects. In contrast, HDL cholesterol levels tend to be lower in NAFLD patients [44].

2.2. Associated metabolic syndrome

In our population, the majority of patients (69%) had a metabolic syndrome. This was in line with several studies [44-46] and underlined the close relationship between NAFLD and metabolic syndrome.

3. Eating habits and survey

3.1. Eating habits

In our study, we found that 86% of our population practiced Ramadan fasting.Indeed, Aliasghari et al showed in their study that Ramadan fasting could be useful in improving NAFLD,by decreasing all anthropometric parameters, fasting glucose, plasma insulin and insulin resistance and reducing inflammation[49].Not all our patients were practicing intermittent fasting or following a ketogenic diet.Several studies have suggested that intermittent fasting may have beneficial effects on NAFLD, by reducing liver fat, improving lipid and carbohydrate metabolism and reducing inflammation [50,51]. In this respect, the study by Drinda et al[52] showed that intermittent fasting reduced NAFLD in 697 participants. After intermittent fasting, there was a decrease in fasting glucose, glycated hemoglobin, body mass index and liver enzymes. In addition, the number of fasting days was positively correlated with an improvement in the hepatic steatosis index.On the other hand, numerous studies have demonstrated that the ketogenic diet has positive effects on NAFLD, improving body weight, liver enzymes and lipid and carbohydrate metabolism [51,53].Furthermore, in our study we found that 57% of patients had had previous education about the Mediterranean diet.However, multiple studies have shown that the Mediterranean diet was associated with a lower likelihood of NAFLD and was the most effective d i e t for treating NAFLD[54,55].In addition, 40% of our patients did not chew their food well. A study carried out in Korea [56] found that fast food was associated with an increased risk of NAFLD in Korean adults.What's more, our study found that 14% of the population ate their meals in restaurants. Indeed, a case-control study by Tavakoli et al, conducted on 100 NAFLD cases and 300 age-matched normal controls, reported that there was a relationship between fast food consumption and NAFLD[57].

3.2.Results of the food survey

3.2.1. Total energy expenditure and intake

Spontaneous caloric intake in our population (3386.14 kcal) was higher than energy requirements (2490.14 kcal). These results are comparable to those found in the literature. Indeed, several studies have demonstrated that subjects with NAFLD have high caloric intakes [58,59].

3.2.2. Intake of macronutrients

•Carbohydrate intake

Mean carbohydrate intake was 336.61 ± 127.74g/d, corresponding to a mean intake of 5.86± 2.22g/kg/d. This intake was excessive and exceeded the WHO recommended carbohydrate standard of 5g/kg/d. A cross-sectional epidemiological study in the USA revealed that excessive carbohydrate consumption was associated with an increased risk of developing non-alcoholic fatty liver disease (NAFLD). In fact, dietary carbohydrates can be converted to fat in the liver, which may have contributed to the development of NAFLD[60].

•Lipid intake

Mean lipid intake was 80.54± 32.17g/d, corresponding to a mean intake of 1.4± 0.58 g/kg/Pi. This intake was excessive and exceeded the WHO recommended lipid standard of 1g/kg/Pi.Hydes et al have shown that an increase in dietary fat increases hepatic fat and thus leads to the development of NAFLD[61].

•Protein intake

Mean protein intake was 78.84± 24.42g/d, corresponding to a mean intake of 1.36± 0.41g/kg/Pi. This intake was very high, and exceeded the WHO recommended protein standards of 0.8 to 1g/kg/Pi. A study carried out in Germany found that proteins played a role in the development and/or progression of NAFLD. Indeed, patients with
NAFLD had a high protein intake[62].

3.2.3. Contribution of SFA, MUFA and PUFA

• AGS contribution

Mean SFA intake was 23 ± 5.5% of TEA, which was excessive and exceeded the recommended standards for SFA < 7% TEA set by the Swiss Federal Office of Public Health (FOPH) and the European Society of Cardiology (ESC). Several studies have found that saturated fatty acids have a detrimental effect on NAFLD, as they contribute to increased liver and visceral fat[63,64].

- **MUFA intake**

The average intake of MUFA was 48.7± 12.67% of TEA, which was excessive and exceeded the recommended standards for MUFA 15% TEA set by the Swiss Federal Office of Public Health (FOPH) and the European Society of Cardiology (ESC). These results concur with those of Cortez-Pinto et al[65]who revealed a high consumption of MUFAs in patients with NAFLD.Similarly, Alferink et al showed in their study that consumption of MUFA did not have a beneficial effect on NAFLD[66]. Furthermore, Sagi et al found no association between MUFA and the development of NAFLD[67]. However, de Wit et al found in their study that could reduce steatosis in patients with NAFLD[68].

- **PUFA intake**

The mean PUFA intake was 28.31 ± 11.87% TEA, which was excessive and exceeded the recommended PUFA6-8% TEA standards of the Swiss Federal Office of Public Health (SFOPH) and the European Society of Cardiology (ESC).According to a study carried out in Spain, polyunsaturated acids were found to play a protective role against non-alcoholic fatty liver disease (NAFLD)[69].On the other hand, the study by Cortez-Pinto et al analyzed PUFA intake, and showed that a lower consumption of n-3 PUFAs and a higher n-6/n-3 ratio have were observed in patients with NAFLD and NASH compared with controls[65].

3.2.4. Cholesterol, sugar and fiber content

- **Cholesterol intake**

Mean dietary cholesterol intake in our population was 115.33± 119.71mg/d. This intake was in line with ANSES recommendations< 300 mg/d.Several studies have reported no significant difference in the levels of cholesterol intake between NAFLD patients and healthy subjects[65,67].While a Japanese study [70]found that cholesterol intake was significantly higher in NAFLD patients than in healthy controls.

•Sugar intake

Average sugar (sucrose) intake in our population was 124.54±

39.68mg/d. This intake exceeded ANSES recommendations< 100 mg/d.

Multiple studies have found that a sucrose-rich diet contributes to the development of NAFLD [71,72].

•Fiber intake

Average sugar intake in our population was 25.6 ± 11.18 mg/d. This intake was below the ANSES recommendation of 30 g/d.Various studies have observed that subjects with NAFLD had diets low in dietary fibre [65,73].Furthermore, a study in the USA reported that an increase in total fibre intake from 38 mg/kg/d to 117 mg/kg/d reduced the risk of NAFLD by 60%, so that a high daily fibre intake was associated with a preventive effect against NAFLD[74].

3.2.5. Micronutrient intake

The results showed that the average intake of vitamin B9, calcium, magnesium and potassium was insufficient in relation to ANSES recommendations. In addition, the average intake of vitamin B1, vitamin C, vitamin E, iron, sodium, zinc and phosphoruscorresponded to the Recommended Dietary Allowances.A study by Pickett-Blakely et al revealed that subjects with NAFLD were deficient in zinc and vitamins A, D and E, and had a high intake of iron [75].Another study by Licata et al showed that patients with NAFLD were deficient in zinc and vitamins A, C, D and group B, and had a high intake of iron [76].Furthermore, a study carried out in Brazil on 72 NAFLD patients found that these patients had a high intake of vitamin C (27%) and selenium (73.6%), in addition to a significant deficiency of vitamin A (98.3%) and vitamin E (100%)[77].

3.3. Frequencies consumption

According to the food frequency questionnaire, we noted that :

- More than ¾ of the population consumed white sugar, white bread and fruits high in fructose such as watermelons, grapes and apricots on a daily basis.
- Around half of our patients consumed fruits daily, which are also very rich in fructose, such as pears, figs, dates and bananas.

- At the same time, we also ensured that no patients consumed decaffeinated coffee and symbiotic yoghurt.
According to several studies, the foods that our patients consume most (white sugar, white bread and fructose-rich fruit) are associated with an increased risk of developing NAFLD[78,79].

On the other hand, numerous studies have shown that foods not consumed by our population (decaffeinated coffee and symbiotic yoghurt) have protective effects for NAFLD[80,81]. A study by Vijay et al [82] showed that NAFLD patients consumed significantly more refined rice, animal fat, red meat, refined sugar and fried foods, and consumed fewer vegetables, fruits and vegetables. legumes, nuts, seeds and milk than controls. Consumption of red meat, animal fat, nuts and refined rice was positively associatedto NAFLD diagnosis and the presence of fibrosis, while consumption of leafy vegetables, fruits and dried legumes was negatively associated. Consumption of fried foods was positively associated with NAFLD, while consumption of boiled foods had a negative association.Furthermore, an Iranian study found that consumption of red meat, fats and sweets was high, while consumption of whole grains, fruits and vegetables was lower in NAFLD patients. Furthermore, there was a positive association between Western diet and the risk of NAFLD, while adherence to the Mediterranean diet was significantly associated with the severity of hepatic steatosis[83].

RECOMMENDATIONS

In the light of our results, we confirm that the most effective process for preventing and treating non-alcoholic fatty liver disease and for achieving good health is through nutrition and health education focusing on a diet compatible with individual dietary preferences and lifestyle habits, regular physical activity and lifestyle modification. We therefore propose the following recommendations:Adapted diet: A diet adapted to NAFLD should include foods that promote liver health and reduce fat accumulation. This may involve reducing consumption of foods high in added sugar, saturated fats and trans fats, as well as avoiding processed foods. Foods such as green leafy vegetables, fish and legumes can be beneficial for liver health.Regular physical activity: In addition to diet, physical activity plays a crucial role in the prevention and treatment of NAFLD. Regular physical activity, adapted to the individual's abilities and preferences, is recommended to promote weight loss, reduce fat accumulation in the liver and improve insulin sensitivity. Exercises such as walking, swimming, cycling, yoga or weight training can be beneficial. Lifestyle modification: To prevent and treat NAFLD, it may be necessary to review certain lifestyle habits. This may include adjustments such as avoiding alcohol consumption, stopping smoking, promoting breast-feeding, managing stress effectively, maintaining a healthy weight, and getting enough sleep.

CONCLUSIONS

Non-Alcoholic Fatty Liver Disease (NAFLD) is a metabolic disease linked to the excessive accumulation of fat (steatosis) in the liver. It is defined by the presence of lipid droplets (steatosis) in more than 5% of hepatocytes without excessive alcohol consumption and after exclusion of all other causes of liver disease.NAFLD comprises a group of liver disorders ranging from simple steatosis to more progressive forms such as non-alcoholic steatohepatitis (NASH), characterized by liver inflammation, and liver fibrosis, can lead to NAFLD-related cirrhosis and hepatocellular carcinoma.Non-alcoholic fatty liver is the most common chronic liver disease worldwide, with a prevalence of almost 25% in the general population.NAFLD is a complex disease whose severity is influenced by genetic, environmental and behavioral factors (such as diet, physical activity and socioeconomic influences). NAFLD is considered the hepatic manifestation of metabolic syndrome and involves pathological changes in several systems, including metabolic diseases (such as metabolic syndrome, type 2 diabetes mellitus, obesity and hypertension), cardiovascular diseases (such as coronary heart disease, atherosclerosis, cardiomyopathy and arrhythmia), extrahepatic carcinomas (such as gastric and colorectal cancer) and chronic kidney disease.In this context, our study focused on describing the dietary and lifestyle habits of patients with NAFLD.To this end, we conducted a descriptive cross-sectional study between November 17, 2022 and February 03, 2023. It involved 42 patients with non-alcoholic fatty liver disease. The patients recruited all consulted the hepato-gastroenterology department of Charles Nicolle Hospital in Tunis.The results of our study showed that the sex ratio M/F was equal to 0.4, 64% of our patients had a low level of education (no schooling or primary schooling), the majority of our patients had an average socioeconomic level, the most frequent history in our population was hypertension (45%).%), dyslipidemia (45%), diabetes (40%). What's more, 45% of our patients are overweight and 55% are obese, while the majority (69%) present a syndrome Metabolic and most of our population (80%) did not have advanced liver fibrosis. In addition, and the majority of women were postmenopausal and had a history of breast-feeding parity.In addition, the main dietary habits found in patients with non-alcoholic fatty liver disease were: a caloric diet, a diet rich in carbohydrates, lipids, proteins, SFAs, MUFAs, PUFAs, sugar (sucrose), fructose-rich fruit and a diet low in fiber. In addition, the main lifestyle habits of our population were sedentary, but smoking was not frequently found in our population. These results are in line with a number of previous studies, which have highlighted the predominance of women, metabolic syndrome, sedentary lifestyle, caloric diet and a diet rich in carbohydrates, lipids and proteins. This study can be seen as a starting point for further work. It would be interesting to complete the study and expand the population size in order to :

➢ Evaluate adherence of subjects with non-alcoholic fatty liver disease to dietary prescriptions and encouragement of long-term physical activity.

REFERENCES

1. Tagkou NM, Goossens N. Nonalcoholic fatty liver disease: diagnosis and treatment in 2022. Schweiz Gastroenterol. March 7, 2023;1-10.

2. Non-alcoholic fatty liver disease (NAFLD/NASH) | SNFGE.org - Société savante French medical journal of hepato-gastroenterology and digestive oncology [Internet]. [cited March 24, 2023]. Available from: https://www.snfge.org/content/steatose-hepatique-non- alcoolique-nafldnash

3. NASH (EASL-2017 recommendations) [Internet]. FMC-HGE. [cited March 24, 2023]. Available from: https://www.fmcgastro.org/texte-postu/postu-2019-paris/nash- recommendations-easl-2017/

4. Hobeika C, Ronot M, Beaufrere A, Paradis V, Soubrane O, Cauchy F. Syndrome metabolism and liver surgery. J Chir Visceral. June 1, 2020;157(3):235-43.

5. Petit J. Application of European recommendations in steatosis screening of type II diabetic patients. 2019;

6. Younossi ZM, Koenig AB, Abdelatif D, Fazel Y, Henry L, Wymer M. Global epidemiology of nonalcoholic fatty liver disease-Meta-analytic assessment of prevalence, incidence, and outcomes. Hepatol Baltim Md. Jul 2016;64(1):73-84.

7. Charlton MR, Burns JM, Pedersen RA, Watt KD, Heimbach JK, Dierkhising RA. Frequency and Outcomes of Liver Transplantation for Nonalcoholic Steatohepatitis in the United States. Gastroenterology. oct 2011;141(4):1249-53.

8. Alberti KGMM, Eckel RH, Grundy SM, Zimmet PZ, Cleeman JI, Donato KA, et al. Harmonizing the metabolic syndrome: a joint interim

statement of the International Diabetes Federation Task Force on Epidemiology and Prevention; National Heart, Lung, and Blood Institute; American Heart Association; World Heart Federation; International Atherosclerosis Society; and International Association for the Study of Obesity. Circulation. 20 Oct 2009;120(16):1640-5.

9. EASL-Guidelines-for-FibroScan_EN.pdf [Internet]. [cited March 22, 2023]. Available from: https://www.echosens.com/wp-content/uploads/2021/07/EASL-Guidelines-for- FibroScan_EN.pdf

10. Bouchoucha M, Akrout M, Bellali H, Bouchoucha R, Tarhouni F, Mansour AB, et al. Development and validation of a food photography manual, as a tool for estimation of food portion size in epidemiological dietary surveys in Tunisia. Libyan J Med. August 31, 2016;11:10.3402/ljm.v11.32676.

11. 9285_rec_nutr_160907_college_valide_pdt_zis_a5_modifie_suite_err atum.pdf [Internet]. [cited 26 Apr 2023]. Available from: https://www.health.belgium.be/sites/default/files/uploads/fields/fpshealth_t heme_file/9285_rec_nutr_160907_college_valide_pdt_zis_a5_modifie_sui te_erratum.pdf

12. Diet, nutrition and the prevention of chronic diseases: report of a WHO/FAO Expert Consultation; [WHO/FAO Expert Consultation on Diet, Nutrition and the Prevention of Chronic Diseases, Geneva, January 28 -]. 1. February 2002]. 2003. 180 p. (WHO Technical Report Series).

13. World Health Organization. Global action plan on physical activity 2018-2030: more active people for a healthier world [Internet]. Geneva: World Health Organization; 2018 [cited 2023 May 6]. 101 p. Available from: https://apps.who.int/iris/handle/10665/272722

14. Cassard-Doulcier AM, Gabriel P. Obesity-related liver inflammation (NASH). Ol Body Fat Lipids. Jan 1, 2011;18.

15. Aleksandrova K, Boeing H, Nöthlings U, Jenab M, Fedirko V, Kaaks

R, et al. Inflammatory and metabolic biomarkers and risk of liver and biliary tract cancer. Hepatol Baltim Md. Sept 2014;60(3):858-71.

16. Yamauchi T, Tobe K, Tamemoto H, Ueki K, Kaburagi Y, Yamamoto-Honda R, et al. Insulin signalling and insulin actions in the muscles and livers of insulin-resistant, insulin receptor substrate 1-deficient mice. Mol Cell Biol. June 1996;16(6):3074-84.

17. Saltiel AR, Kahn CR. Insulin signalling and the regulation of glucose and lipid.metabolism. Nature. Dec 13 2001;414(6865):799-806.

18. Jornayvaz FR, Samuel VT, Shulman GI. The role of muscle insulin resistance in the pathogenesis of atherogenic dyslipidemia and nonalcoholic fatty liver disease associated with the metabolic syndrome. Annu Rev Nutr. August 21, 2010;30:273-90.

19. Leite NC, Villela-Nogueira CA, Cardoso CRL, Salles GF. Non-alcoholic fatty liver disease and diabetes: From physiopathological interplay to diagnosis and treatment. World J Gastroenterol WJG. 14 Jul 2014;20(26):8377-92.

20. Anty R, Gual P. Pathophysiology of metabolic hepatic steatosis. Presse Médicale. Dec 2019;48(12):1468-83.

21. Brunt EM, Kleiner DE, Carpenter DH, Rinella M, Harrison SA, Loomba R, et al. NAFLD: Reporting Histologic Findings in Clinical Practice. Hepatol Baltim Md. May 2021;73(5):2028-38.

22. Jackson KG, Way GW, Zhou H. Bile acids and sphingolipids in non-alcoholic fatty liver disease. Chin Med J (Engl). 20 May 2022;135(10):1163-71.

23. Değertekin B, Tözün N, Demir F, Söylemez G, Parkan Ş, Gürtay E, et al. The Changing Prevalence of Non-Alcoholic Fatty Liver Disease (NAFLD) in Turkey in the Last Decade. Turk J Gastroenterol. March 1, 2021;32(3):302-12.

24. Hu X, Huang Y, Bao Z, Wang Y, Shi D, Liu F, et al. Prevalence and

factors associated with nonalcoholic fatty liver disease in shanghai work-units. BMC Gastroenterol. 14 Sep 2012;12:123.

25. Nagral A, Bangar M, Menezes S, Bhatia S, Butt N, Ghosh J, et al. Gender Differences in Nonalcoholic Fatty Liver Disease. Euroasian J Hepato-Gastroenterol. Jul 2022;12(Suppl 1):S19-25.

26. Chen XY, Wang C, Huang YZ, Zhang LL. Nonalcoholic fatty liver disease shows significant sex dimorphism. World J Clin Cases. Feb 16, 2022;10(5):1457-72.

27. Yang YJ, Kim T, Hong YP. Urinary Phthalate Levels Associated with the Risk of Nonalcoholic Fatty Liver Disease in Adults: The Korean National Environmental Health Survey (KoNEHS) 2012-2014. Int J Environ Res Public Health. jan 2021;18(11):6035.

28. Motamed N, Maadi M, Sohrabi M, Keyvani H, Poustchi H, Zamani F. Rural Residency has a Protective Effect and Marriage is a Risk Factor for NAFLD. Hepat Mon [Internet]. 2016 [cited May 21, 2023];16(7). Available from: https://brieflands.com/articles/hepatmon-15656.html#abstract

29. Vilar-Gomez E, Nephew LD, Vuppalanchi R, Gawrieh S, Mladenovic A, Pike F, et al. High-quality diet, physical activity, and college education are associated with low risk of NAFLD among the US population. Hepatology. June 2022;75(6):1491.

30. Zarean E, Goujani R, Rahimian G, Ahamdi A. Prevalence and risk factors of non- alcoholic fatty liver disease in southwest Iran: a population-based case-control study. Clin Exp Hepatol. Sept 2019;5(3):224-31.

31. Hu W, Liu Z, Hao H rong, Yu W nan, Wang X qing, Shao X juan, et al. Correlation between income and non-alcoholic fatty liver disease in a Chinese population. Ann Endocrinol. Dec 2020;81(6):561-6.

32. Li Z, Xue J, Chen P, Chen L, Yan S, Liu L. Prevalence of

nonalcoholic fatty liver disease in mainland of China: A meta-analysis of published studies: Prevalence of nonalcoholic fatty liver disease. J Gastroenterol Hepatol. Jan 2014;29(1):42-51.

33. Nabi O. Nonalcoholic fatty liver disease in France, epidemiology and prognosis: analysis of data from the Constances cohort and the Système National des Données de Santé (SNDS) [Internet][phdthesis]. Sorbonne University; 2022 [cited 2023 May 24]. Available from: https://theses.hal.science/tel-03827839

34. Ameur FZ, Ben Amor S, Ghannei O, Ben Mansour W, Ben Chaaben N, Safer L. Prevalence of type 2 diabetes in patients with nonalcoholic fatty liver disease. Ann Endocrinol. Oct 1, 2021;82(5):506.

35. Armandi A, Bugianesi E. Extrahepatic Outcomes of Nonalcoholic Fatty Liver Disease: Cardiovascular Diseases. Clin Liver Dis. May 1, 2023;27(2):239-50.

36. Wang J, Wu AH, Stanczyk FZ, Porcel J, Noureddin M, Terrault NA, et al. Associations Between Reproductive and Hormone-Related Factors and Risk of Nonalcoholic Fatty Liver Disease in a Multiethnic Population. Clin Gastroenterol Hepatol. June 1, 2021;19(6):1258-1266.e1.

37. Park Y, Sinn DH, Oh JH, Goh MJ, Kim K, Kang W, et al. The Association Between Breastfeeding and Nonalcoholic Fatty Liver Disease in Parous Women: A Nation-wide Cohort Study. Hepatology. Dec 2021;74(6):2988-97.

38. Völzke H, Schwarz S, Baumeister SE, Wallaschofski H, Schwahn C, Grabe HJ, et al. Menopausal status and hepatic steatosis in a general female population. Gut. 1 Apr 2007;56(4):594-5.

39. Jung HS, Chang Y, Kwon MJ, Sung E, Yun KE, Cho YK, et al. Smoking and the Risk of Non-Alcoholic Fatty Liver Disease: A Cohort Study. Am J Gastroenterol. March 2019;114(3):453-63.

40. Jarvis H, O'Keefe H, Craig D, Stow D, Hanratty B, Anstee QM. Does moderate alcohol consumption accelerate the progression of liver disease in NAFLD? A systematic review and narrative synthesis. BMJ Open. Jan 2022;12(1):e049767.

41. Hallsworth K, Thoma C, Moore S, Ploetz T, Anstee QM, Taylor R, et al. Non-alcoholic fatty liver disease is associated with higher levels of objectively measured sedentary behaviour and lower levels of physical activity than matched healthy controls. Frontline Gastroenterol. Jan 1, 2015;6(1):44-51.

42. Khoonsari M, Mohammad Hosseini Azar M, Ghavam R, Hatami K, Asobar M, Gholami A, et al. Clinical Manifestations and Diagnosis of Nonalcoholic Fatty Liver Disease. Iran J Pathol. 2017;12(2):99-105.

43. Milić S, Lulić D, Štimac D. Non-alcoholic fatty liver disease and obesity: Biochemical, metabolic and clinical presentations. World J Gastroenterol WJG. 28 Jul.2014;20(28):9330-7.

44. Shen J, Chan HLY, Wong GLH, Choi PCL, Chan AWH, Chan HY, et al. Non-invasive diagnosis of non-alcoholic steatohepatitis by combined serum biomarkers. J Hepatol.June 2012;56(6):1363-70.

45. Cuthbertson DJ, Irwin A, Sprung VS, Jones H, Pugh CJA, Daousi C, et al. Ectopic lipid storage in non-alcoholic fatty liver disease is not mediated by impaired mitochondrial oxidative capacity in skeletal muscle. Clin Sci. Dec 1, 2014;127(12):655-63.

46. Cabrera D, Moncayo-Rizzo J, Cevallos K, Alvarado-Villa G. Waist Circumference as a Risk Factor for Non-Alcoholic Fatty Liver Disease in Older Adults in Guayaquil, Ecuador. Geriatrics. Apr 14, 2023;8(2):42.

47. Kim YC, Cho YK, Lee WY, Kim HJ, Park JH, Park DI, et al. Serum adipocyte-specific fatty acid-binding protein is associated with nonalcoholic fatty liver disease in apparently healthy subjects. J Nutr Biochem. March 2011;22(3):289-92.

48. Kalhan SC, Guo L, Edmison J, Dasarathy S, McCullough AJ, Hanson RW, et al. Plasma metabolomic profile in nonalcoholic fatty liver disease. Metabolism. March 2011;60(3):404-13.

49. Aliasghari F, Izadi A, Gargari BP, Ebrahimi S. The Effects of Ramadan Fasting on Body Composition, Blood Pressure, Glucose Metabolism, and Markers of Inflammation in NAFLD Patients: An Observational Trial. J Am Coll Nutr. 17 Nov 2017;36(8):640-5.

50. Semmler G, Datz C, Trauner M. Eating, diet, and nutrition for the treatment of non-responsiveness.alcoholic fatty liver disease. Clin Mol Hepatol. Dec 14, 2022;29(Suppl):S244-60.

51. Ristic-Medic D, Bajerska J, Vucic V. Crosstalk between dietary patterns, obesity and nonalcoholic fatty liver disease. World J Gastroenterol. 21 Jul 2022;28(27):3314-33.

52. Drinda S, Grundler F, Neumann T, Lehmann T, Steckhan N, Michalsen A, et al. Effects of Periodic Fasting on Fatty Liver Index-A Prospective Observational Study. Nutrients. 30 Oct 2019;11(11):2601.

53. Sripongpun P, Churuangsuk C, Bunchorntavakul C. Current Evidence Concerning Effects of Ketogenic Diet and Intermittent Fasting in Patients with Nonalcoholic Fatty Liver. J Clin Transl Hepatol. August 28, 2022;10(4):730-9.

54. George ES, Georgousopoulou EN, Mellor DD, Chrysohoou C, Pitsavos C, Panagiotakos DB. Exploring the Path of Mediterranean Diet, Non-Alcoholic Fatty Liver Disease.(NAFLD) and Inflammation towards 10-Year Cardiovascular Disease (CVD) Risk: The ATTICA Study 10-Year Follow-Up (2002-2012). Nutrients. Jan 2022;14(12):2367.

55. Katsagoni CN, Papatheodoridis GV, Ioannidou P, Deutsch M, Alexopoulou A, Papadopoulos N, et al. Improvements in clinical characteristics of patients with non-alcoholic fatty liver disease, after an intervention based on the Mediterranean lifestyle: a randomised

controlled clinical trial. Br J Nutr. Jul 2018;120(2):164-75.

56. Lee S, Ko BJ, Gong Y, Han K, Lee A, Han BD, et al. Self-reported eating speed in relation to non-alcoholic fatty liver disease in adults. Eur J Nutr. 1 Feb 2016;55(1):327-33.

57. Tavakoli HR, Rahmati-Najarkolaei F, Malkami A, Dizavi AR. The relation between fast food consumption and nonalcoholic fatty liver: A case-control study. Iran J Endocrinol Metab. 2018;20(1):22-30.

58. Aktary ML, Eller LK, Nicolucci AC, Reimer RA. Cross-sectional analysis of the health profile and dietary intake of a sample of Canadian adults diagnosed with non-alcoholic fatty liver disease. Food Nutr Res. 18 Sep 2020;64:10.29219/fnr.v64.4548.

59. Sathiaraj E, Chutke M, Reddy MY, Pratap N, Rao PN, Reddy DN, et al. A case-control study on nutritional risk factors in non-alcoholic fatty liver disease in Indian population. Eur J Clin Nutr. Apr 2011;65(4):533-7.

60. Neuschwander-Tetri BA. Carbohydrate intake and nonalcoholic fatty liver disease: Curr Opin Clin Nutr Metab Care. july 2013;16(4):446-52.

61. Hydes T, Alam U, Cuthbertson DJ. The Impact of Macronutrient Intake on Non- alcoholic Fatty Liver Disease (NAFLD): Too Much Fat, Too Much Carbohydrate, or Just Too Many Calories? Front Nutr. Feb 16, 2021;8:640557.

62. Lang S, Martin A, Farowski F, Wisplinghoff H, Vehreschild MJGT, Liu J, et al. High Protein Intake Is Associated With Histological Disease Activity in Patients With NAFLD. Hepatol Commun. March 26, 2020;4(5):681-95.

63. Lombardi R, Iuculano F, Pallini G, Fargion S, Fracanzani AL. Nutrients, Genetic Factors, and Their Interaction in Non-Alcoholic Fatty Liver Disease and Cardiovascular Disease. Int J Mol Sci. 19 Nov 2020;21(22):8761.

64. Della Pepa G, Vetrani C, Lombardi G, Bozzetto L, Annuzzi G,

Rivellese AA. Isocaloric Dietary Changes and Non-Alcoholic Fatty Liver Disease in High Cardiometabolic Risk Individuals. Nutrients. 26 Sep 2017;9(10):1065.

65. Cortez-Pinto H, Jesus L, Barros H, Lopes C, Moura MC, Camilo ME. How different is the dietary pattern in non-alcoholic steatohepatitis patients? Clin Nutr Edinb Scotl. Oct 2006;25(5):816-23.

66. Alferink LJ, Kiefte-de Jong JC, Erler NS, Veldt BJ, Schoufour JD, de Knegt RJ, et al. Association of dietary macronutrient composition and non-alcoholic fatty liver disease in an ageing population: the Rotterdam Study. Gut. June 2019;68(6):1088-98.

67. Zelber-Sagi S, Nitzan-Kaluski D, Goldsmith R, Webb M, Blendis L, Halpern Z, et al. Long term nutritional intake and the risk for non-alcoholic fatty liver disease (NAFLD): a population based study. J Hepatol. Nov 2007;47(5):711-7.

68. de Wit NJW, Afman LA, Mensink M, Müller M. Phenotyping the effect of diet on non alcoholic fatty liver disease. J Hepatol. dec 2012;57(6):1370-3.

69. Vancells Lujan P, Viñas Esmel E, Sacanella Meseguer E. Overview of Non-Alcoholic Fatty Liver Disease (NAFLD) and the Role of Sugary Food Consumption and Other Dietary Components in Its Development. Nutrients. Apr 24, 2021;13(5):1442.

70. Yasutake K, Nakamuta M, Shima Y, Ohyama A, Masuda K, Haruta N, et al. Nutritional investigation of non-obese patients with non-alcoholic fatty liver disease: the significance of dietary cholesterol. Scand J Gastroenterol. 2009;44(4):471-7.

71. Nier A, Brandt A, Conzelmann IB, Özel Y, Bergheim I. Non-Alcoholic Fatty Liver Disease in Overweight Children: Role of Fructose Intake and Dietary Pattern. Nutrients. 19 Sep 2018;10(9):1329.

72. Ishimoto T, Lanaspa MA, Rivard CJ, Roncal-Jimenez CA, Orlicky DJ,

Cicerchi C, et al. High Fat and High Sucrose (Western) Diet Induce Steatohepatitis that is Dependent on Fructokinase. Hepatol Baltim Md. Nov 2013;58(5):1632-43.

73. Wehmeyer MH, Zyriax BC, Jagemann B, Roth E, Windler E, Schulze zur Wiesch J, et al. Nonalcoholic fatty liver disease is associated with excessive calorie intake rather than a distinctive dietary pattern. Medicine (Baltimore). June 10, 2016;95(23):e3887.

74. Zhao H, Yang A, Mao L, Quan Y, Cui J, Sun Y. Association Between Dietary Fiber Intake and Non-alcoholic Fatty Liver Disease in Adults. Front Nutr. 19 Nov 2020;7:593735.

75. Pickett-Blakely O, Young K, Carr RM. Micronutrients in Nonalcoholic Fatty Liver Disease Pathogenesis. Cell Mol Gastroenterol Hepatol. August 23, 2018;6(4):451-62.

76. Licata A, Zerbo M, Como S, Cammilleri M, Soresi M, Montalto G, et al. The Role of Vitamin Deficiency in Liver Disease: To Supplement or Not Supplement? Nutrients. 10 Nov 2021;13(11):4014.

77. Coelho JM, Cansanção K, Perez R de M, Leite NC, Padilha P, Ramalho A, et al. Association between serum and dietary antioxidant micronutrients and advanced liver fibrosis in non-alcoholic fatty liver disease: an observational study. PeerJ. 17 Sep 2020;8:e9838.

78. Coronati M, Baratta F, Pastori D, Ferro D, Angelico F, Del Ben M. Added Fructose in Non-Alcoholic Fatty Liver Disease and in Metabolic Syndrome: A Narrative Review. Nutrients. March 8, 2022;14(6):1127.

79. Pixner T, Stummer N, Schneider AM, Lukas A, Gramlinger K, Julian V, et al. The Role of Macronutrients in the Pathogenesis, Prevention and Treatment of Non-Alcoholic Fatty Liver Disease (NAFLD) in the Paediatric Population-A Review. Life. June 5, 2022;12(6):839.

80. Brandt A, Nier A, Jin CJ, Baumann A, Jung F, Ribas V, et al. Consumption of decaffeinated coffee protects against the development

of early non-alcoholic steatohepatitis: Role of intestinal barrier function. Redox Biol. Feb 2019;21:101092.

81. Suárez M, Boqué N, del Bas JM, Mayneris-Perxachs J, Arola L, Caimari A. Mediterranean Diet and Multi-Ingredient-Based Interventions for the Management of Non-Alcoholic Fatty Liver Disease. Nutrients. 22 Sep 2017;9(10):1052.

82. Vijay A, Al-Awadi A, Chalmers J, Balakumaran L, Grove JI, Valdes AM, et al. Development of Food Group Tree-Based Analysis and Its Association with Non- Alcoholic Fatty Liver Disease (NAFLD) and Co-Morbidities in a South Indian Population: A Large Case-Control Study. Nutrients. 8 Jul 2022;14(14):2808.

83. MIRMIRAN P, AMIRHAMIDI Z, EJTAHED HS, BAHADORAN Z, AZIZI F.Relationship between Diet and Non-alcoholic Fatty Liver Disease: A Review Article.Iran J Public Health. august 2017;46(8):1007-17.

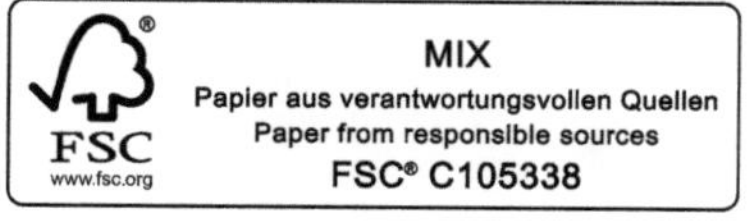

Printed by Books on Demand GmbH, Norderstedt / Germany